HEALING THE GUT

A Crib Sheet for Eliminating SIBO

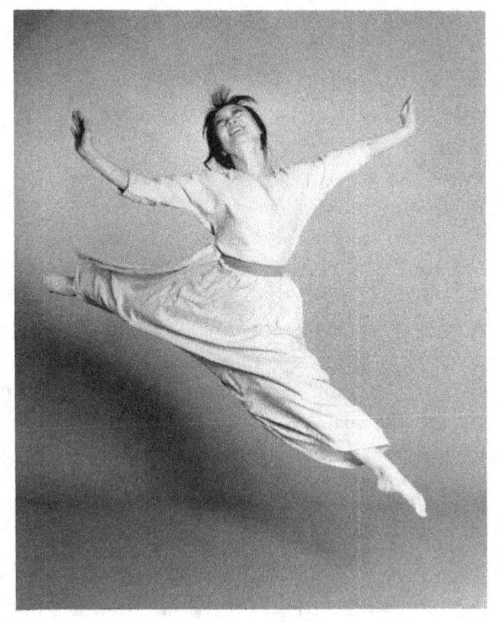

SHEPHERD HOODWIN

HEALING THE GUT
A Crib Sheet for Eliminating SIBO

Summerjoy Press
99 Pearl
Laguna Niguel CA 92677-4818

shoodwin@gmail.com
https://shepherdhoodwin.com

ISBN: 9798664495799

Photograph of Shepherd Hoodwin by John Kilis.
Thank you to Yung Yung Lerner for the photo of her dancing.

Dedicated to

Wade Binley, D.C.

&

Glenn Frieder, D.C.

INTRODUCTION

I've had sluggish digestion and a bloated stomach all my life but I never thought that something was seriously wrong with my gut. However, with various strategies for solving other health issues not working, my chiropractor and nutritional counselor, Wade Binley, asked me to get a hydrogen breath test. It turned out I had SIBO (Small Intestinal Bacterial Overgrowth). He prescribed a rigorous diet and regimen to heal my gut, pointing me to some online resources.

Trying to figure out what I was supposed to do made my brain hurt. There's a great deal of information out there but it's mostly not presented clearly for the beginner. I felt so overwhelmed by details that I couldn't see the big picture. As I finally figured it out, I thought I could save others some trouble by presenting this distillation. I've drawn ideas from a variety of sources and added some of my own; I'm sure you will, too.

Shepherd Hoodwin
July 7, 2020

CONTENTS

CONTENTS

1 • THE SPECIFIC CARBOHYDRATE DIET (SCD)

SIBO

SIBO—Small Intestinal Bacterial Overgrowth—indicates that the small intestine is damaged. There are a lot of possible causes, such as repeated stomach flus. Once damaged, its ability to absorb nutrition is compromised, so carbohydrates are more likely to stay in it and ferment, feeding bacteria. (Unlike the colon, the small intestine isn't supposed to have a lot of bacteria, whether good or bad). When bad bacteria overgrow, they give out toxins that further damage the membrane. It's a vicious cycle.

It's likely that SIBO is a factor in a number of digestive diseases. There is an epidemic of them today due to our degraded food supply, with GMOs, artificial ingredients, insecticides, and other pollutants that our body doesn't recognize or know what to do with. It's now theorized that the particular dominant strain of bad bacteria that has overgrown determines the particular disease that results; for example, one for Crohn's, another for ulcerative colitis.

SIBO can also contribute to obesity. A fascinating recent news story told of a formerly thin woman who received a fecal implant from an otherwise healthy but obese donor, and she became obese, too.

I wonder whether SIBO contributes to my GERD (acid reflux), as the gas created by the fermentation rises up and pushes open the esophageal valve. Gastroenterologists seem to look only at the stomach.

My symptoms have abated since I've been on this protocol.

SIBO can also be a factor in many conditions that don't obviously concern the gut, such as insomnia and some forms of autism, and mental health issues such as depression. I have a friend who links her periodic depression with bloating. Everything in the body and mind is connected to everything else, which is why a holistic approach to health is essential.

The most definitive way to determine whether you have SIBO is to get a hydrogen breath test, although if you have bloating, a lot of gas, and other digestive problems, there's a good chance that you do.

HEALING THROUGH DIET

A diet was developed starting in the 1920s called SCD—the Specific Carbohydrate Diet—that has had great success in healing SIBO (although the term SIBO is relatively recent) by starving the bacteria so that the small intestine can heal. The bible for SCD is *Breaking the Vicious Cycle* (*BTVC*) by Elaine Gottschall:

http://tinyurl.com/ndsdd3p

It has sold over a million copies since 1994, and there are numerous sites for SCD. According to Gottschall, it has cured many people with Crohn's, celiac, IBS, diverticulitis, and ulcerative colitis. Results are better with children, but many adults have also found that if they stay on SCD for a year after their symptoms have stopped, they can return to a regular healthy diet—their small intestine will then be normal. People with a genetic inability to digest certain foods such as gluten or dairy will probably still need to avoid them, but they won't have the devastating, unpredictable reactions to a wide variety of foods that they'd had previously. I wish more people knew about this. Patients are not likely to hear about dietary cures from their physicians, but instead are just given more medications, which sometimes aggravate their condition. Even gastroenterologists can be surprisingly disinterested in diet.

The small intestine is not needed to digest monosaccharides, or single sugars, such as fruit and honey. The main thrust of SCD is to eliminate all other carbohydrates—disaccharides and polysaccharides—that *do* require digestion in the small intestine: most particularly, grains, sugar, and starchy vegetables such as potatoes. The idea is to make digestion as easy as possible in order to let the small intestine rest while it heals.

SCD is similar to the Paleo and GAPS diets, but it also eliminates some other foods that might be problematic with SIBO, such as those containing immune boosters, since you're trying to calm down your immune system.

FODMAPS

Most non-starchy fruits and vegetables are allowed on SCD. However, recent research has identified something called high FODMAPs, which are carbs that either ferment quickly and/or draw water into the intestines. Some people are more sensitive to them than others, but reducing or eliminating high FODMAP foods when eating meals with animal products, especially, accelerates healing. Animal products digest particularly slowly and slow down the digestion of other foods eaten with them. Beans and nuts also digest more slowly than vegetables and fruit. High FODMAP foods might be fine in small quantities but a problem in larger ones. Eliminating them entirely while on SCD would leave you with little to eat. Instead, try to eat them alone on an empty stomach and let them fully digest before eating heavier foods (typically about half an hour for fruits and an hour for vegetables—I discuss food combining principles below.) This chart shows FODMAPS from low to high:

http://tinyurl.com/SIBOFODMAP

Some foods are on both the low and high FODMAP lists but in different quantities. For example, two Brussels sprouts are low FODMAP, whereas six are high. It's absurd to think of eating only two Brussels sprouts as a side dish unless it's part of mixed vegetables. Instead, have as many as you want on an empty stomach and wait an hour before your main course if that's doable for you.

OTHER PROBLEMATIC FOODS

Some people have trouble with other substances, such as nightshade vegetables (tomatoes, potatoes, peppers, etc.) or high-phenol foods (such as darker fruits), which are a problem with those with leaky gut, and cutting out or limiting those as well might be helpful. As with FODMAPS, eliminating everything you might possibly be sensitive to would leave you with little to eat. SCD is an unusual diet in that, although there are forbidden ("illegal") foods, there's also a wide range of gray-area foods that you personally may or may not react to, so you customize it for your body and continually test new foods.

INTRO DIET

You start with an Intro diet that contains very few foods. It's hoped that you won't react to any of them, but some people react even to this relatively safe list. If your symptoms don't subside within a few days on the Intro diet, you need to eliminate still more foods until you're symptom-free. If you already know you have trouble with some of the foods, don't include them (for example, eggs, dairy, or gelatin). Elaine's Intro diet contains a lot of lactose-free dairy, such as dry curd cottage cheese (which is hard to find, but my Sprouts Farmers Market has it in their deli), but so many people have trouble with even lactose-free dairy that SCD Lifestyle (discussed below) offers a non-dairy version of the Intro diet. It consists mostly of meats, a simple homemade chicken soup, stewed carrots, and grape juice gelatin for snacks. You could also do a raw juice cleanse as your Intro if you tolerate it well.

ADDING BACK FOODS

It's amazing that some people's longtime symptoms can be gone within as little as a day after cutting out their reactive foods. Once your symptoms have subsided, you start adding back foods and see whether they return. For someone with severe issues, it's wise to add only one food back every three days (which is usually long enough for a reaction to surface). If your symptoms are mild, it might be enough to add back one class of foods at a time. For example, someone with severe issues might test butternut squash for three days, then acorn squash, etc. But with mild issues, you might simply test all squash, summer and winter, and add it back into your diet if you don't have a problem. (Squash, like carrots, are foods that few people have trouble with.) Since my case isn't severe, I didn't necessarily wait three days to add back in another new food I was confident in. If your case is severe, you'll want to be more cautious, because you want to be able to identify exactly what you're reacting to.

A sensitivity may be either temporary or permanent, so if you react to something, you might test it again later when you've healed further unless you experienced anaphylactic shock (a very severe allergic reaction). A few days after starting SCD, I reacted to raw juice, but a week later, I didn't.

Especially if you have a severe case, don't assume that you don't react to something just because you weren't aware of it being problematic earlier. A reaction might have been masked by stronger reactions to other things. Once you've eliminated those other things, you might find that this food is problematic, too. Test everything if you want to be on the safe side.

I went through the ebook *SCD Lifestyle: From Surviving to Thriving* (discussed below) and chose these low-FODMAP foods to add back into meals after the Intro diet, and wrote them into my calendar in this order:

Butternut squash, acorn squash, bananas, pineapple (stewed—it's fibrous), spinach, zucchini, raw vegetable/fruit juice, green beans, cantaloupe*, nut milk yogurt, cabbage, peas, beets, broccoli, olives, papaya, blueberries, and lentils.

* I probably could have handled cantaloupe raw right away, since it's not fibrous, but to be on the safe side, I roasted it, tossed with a little honey, using a simple recipe I found online. It was delicious. I almost never cook fruit so it was an interesting change.

I ended up adding in some high FODMAP foods early on, too, such as pureed cauliflower, but ate them before meals. I didn't have any problems with them.

HOMEMADE FOODS

Almost everything must be homemade because packaged goods often have added illegal ingredients (and don't necessarily reveal all their ingredients, or use different names for illegal foods that you don't recognize). For example, sugar might be added to apple juice but not mentioned on the label (apple cider is usually okay). Manufacturing practices change constantly, and what was safe earlier may not be now. If you are doing SCD with dairy, you make your own yogurt and ferment it for twenty-four hours to eliminate all lactose, rather than the normal four to eight hours. (You can also make vegan yogurt.) When you do buy packaged foods or take supplements and medications, it's important to read labels like a hawk, especially if you're highly sensitive.

LEGAL BUT INTRODUCED CAUTIOUSLY

Some legal foods are only introduced later, and

gradually, as you've healed more. Some kinds of beans are allowed later on (but not soy or chickpeas). Most nuts are fine later on but you have to be more cautious with seeds, since they're more fibrous and might irritate your intestinal membrane while it's trying to heal. Hard-to-digest/highly fibrous foods such as cabbage should wait until you've largely healed unless you juice it or cook it well and puree it. Raw foods can be a problem in the beginning because their fiber is harsher, especially coarse raw vegetables. Some people can't tolerate any raw food at the beginning, whereas others can handle foods such as baby greens or watery fruits such as melons, whose fiber isn't as rough. Raw, very ripe bananas are the one raw food almost everyone can handle at the beginning.

Before SCD, I was eating large raw salads and green smoothies most days. More than half my diet was raw, and I didn't think it was a problem, but no doubt it was contributing to my gas and bloating. Raw foods are perhaps the healthiest foods *if* your small intestine is sound, but otherwise they're difficult. I tried to reintroduce big salads too soon on SCD and immediately had a lot of gas, so I had to back off.

BREAKING DOWN FIBER

Cooking things for a long time is one way to break down the fiber. Pureeing them is another, especially in a high-speed blender such as the Vitamix. (Costco has the best prices I've seen on powerful blenders. If you're not a member, you can still buy from their site with a surcharge.) If you have severe symptoms, at first you'll probably be eating a lot of well-cooked and pureed vegetables reminiscent of baby food. However, early on I added back green smoothies with vegetables that don't have tough fiber, such as chard and baby greens; even without cooking them, blending them well breaks down their fiber to some degree. It's worth testing.

Costco and other stores sell large bags of organic "Power Greens" that combine baby kale, spinach, and chard. That's my smoothie staple, along with one-pound boxes of baby salad greens that I also use for salads.

Raw vegetable and fruit juices exclude most of the fiber and are especially worth trying early. They are nutritional powerhouses, full of vitamins and minerals, and raw foods have enzymes, which are lacking in cooked food. (It's recommended that you dilute them with water fifty-fifty, since they're so concentrated.) Even if the whole fruits and vegetables are high FODMAP, that probably isn't as much an issue when the fiber is removed. Still, it's a good idea to drink juices on an empty stomach away from a heavy meal since they digest quickly.

REASONS FOR EXCLUDING FOODS

The main reason a food is SCD illegal is that it contains starches. When there are other reasons, the resources sometimes tell you their reasoning and may acknowledge that they're not sure whether they need to be excluded but would rather be safe than sorry.

An example is Pau d'Arco tea. Elaine wrote, "I would not advise other SCDers to use the bark tea because I do not fully understand its action. You know me, if I don't know for sure, don't do it." Another commenter wrote, "It contains steroidal saponins, and is both an immune booster and a laxative. It is not allowed on SCD." (Many people with digestive disorders have diarrhea, so they need to avoid laxatives.) However, Wade prescribed it as part of my antibiotic protocol (below), so I used it.

Some foods have migrated from legal to illegal, or vice-versa, over the years. Some fermented soy products were legal, but Elaine felt that people were overdoing them and made them illegal. (I decided to go with her original advice and am using small amounts of organic gluten-free Tamari and miso.) Stevia was prohibited earlier, but now small amounts are allowed.

Soy is illegal for various reasons, but I don't completely agree with its vilification. Commercial soybeans, like corn, are usually GMO, which everyone should avoid, but organic foods are non-GMO by definition. Soybeans contain enzyme inhibitors that can block protein digestion and a clot-promoting substance, but they are mostly eliminated after fermenting and/or sprouting, as with miso, or tofu made from sprouted soybeans (which is now widely available, such as at Trader Joe's). Many fermented soy products also contain gluten, but not all.

Many things in health aren't black and white—you have to weigh the pros and cons. With some things, even a small amount might set you off; others depend on how much you consume. We all need to think for ourselves and test things, seeing how we do with them. I decided that a few organic dried cranberries in my salads would cause no problems, despite having a tiny amount of sugar. I use Trocomare organic seasoning salt, which has kelp as its last ingredient. Seaweed is SCD illegal, but it's in Trocomare in such trace amounts that I'm not concerned about it. Elaine urged fanatical adherence to the diet. It's better to be on the safe side, especially if you're highly sensitive, but when you know what you react to and the reasoning behind each exclusion, you can take a more nuanced approach to SCD. The main thing is not to feed bad bacteria with disaccharides and polysaccharides that you can't yet digest.

Many foods have elements that would be toxic on their own but as part of a whole food, work synergistically with other elements and are not harmful. So just because a toxic chemical can be isolated in a food, it doesn't mean it will hurt you when eaten in moderation in its natural state. In smoothies, I use whole apples, including the seeds. They have trace amounts of arsenic but I'm not convinced that they're a problem.

The SCD legal/illegal foods lists haven't been updated since Elaine died in 2005, so there are some foods whose legality are debated. Without knowing their complete chemical composition, it's hard to make an evaluation based on science. For example, I thought that coconut aminos would be a good tamari substitute. It's legal for GAPS. However, it's debated in the SCD community. An argument against it is that it's made from the tree's sap (not the fruit), and maple syrup, also from sap, is illegal. However, SCDLifestyle.com has a link for purchasing it, so it's probably fine for most people. The best advice is to try it and see whether you react to it.

VEGETARIAN SCD

Many SCDers eat a lot of meat, although Elaine cautions not to overdo it (and it's not necessary to do so). A vegan could not do this diet successfully, but a vegetarian who eats eggs and can tolerate lactose-free milk could pull it off.

POOR BOWEL MOVEMENTS

Until you're able to add back in more fiber, including some raw food, you're likely to get constipated or have otherwise poor bowel movements. That's not good, because you're killing a lot of microbes that you want to get out of your body. You can increase your fruit intake (such as prune juice for constipation) but you don't want to overdo sugar. Magnesium might help. Your best bet is probably to increase cooked vegetables and not eat a lot of meat, which can be constipating. Also consider getting colonic hydrotherapy or giving yourself enemas until your bowel movements are normal.

"CHEATING"

One bad reaction can be a major setback, so it's best not to "cheat" and eat any foods you might react to.

WEIGHT LOSS

You will likely lose weight on this diet, as with most low-carb diets. If you need to, that's great. If you don't, there are ways to minimize weight loss outlined in some of the resources below, such as increasing your fat intake if you can digest fats. If you have trouble digesting fats, try a digestive enzyme that includes lipase.

CHANGES I'VE EXPERIENCED

When I started SCD, my body shifted into a different mode and at first, I was hardly hungry. I lost ten pounds in two weeks. It's like my gut shut down for repairs. After that, my appetite returned to about normal and my weight loss slowed down a great deal. I've always had a sweet tooth but haven't experienced many cravings since I started.

The most unexpected benefit of SCD so far for me is that before SCD, I was often thirsty and drank a great deal of water but it largely passed through me—I was constantly going to the bathroom. Now, that has normalized and I have better hydration.

My number one issue is chronic insomnia, and I undertook SCD hoping that that would be the answer that has eluded me my whole life. So far, I am waking up less during the night and the quality of sleep is generally better, especially when my gut is calm, although I am not yet sleeping more hours. My burping and gas are much reduced but not yet eliminated. After a year on SCD, I have less bloating than I ever recall having, leading me to believe that I must have had SIBO since early childhood. I don't have a flat stomach—it's slightly rounded—but it is no longer distended. I'm looking forward to seeing how this progresses.

AFTER THE DIET

Some people need (or prefer) to stay on SCD for many years, but most will eventually be able to go off it.

Since I don't have celiac, I don't intend to stay off all wheat forever, but modern American wheat is problematic. That's possibly because of the Roundup herbicide generously sprayed on it in the U.S.; people who react badly to American wheat sometimes find they have no problem in Europe, where Roundup isn't used. It might also have to do with the issue raised in the book *Wheat Belly*: hybrids developed since 1940 have greatly increased gliadin, a component of gluten. In any case, I'll mostly stick with organic heritage varieties such as spelt, emmer, and faro, or organic sprouted grain breads such as Food for Life Ezekiel 4:9 Bread, which is widely available. Like fermenting, sprouting transforms a food's chemical properties.

SCD is in some ways the opposite of what I thought a healthy diet should be. I tried to eat more than half raw foods, with whole grains, etc., and not much in the way of animal products. SCD isn't an unhealthy diet if you stick with organic, real foods, but it's quite limited at first. (You'll probably want to take some supplements.) However, my former ultra-healthy diet wasn't doing me as much good as it could have because with my damaged gut, I wasn't absorbing all of what I was eating. So first things first: heal the gut, then go back to more fibrous raw foods and some whole grains

2 • RESOURCES FOR THE DIET

SCD LIFESTYLE

http://scdlifestyle.com

belongs to Jordan Reasoner and Steve Wright, who struggled to use *BTVC* to heal themselves and came up with helpful elaborations through their own trial and error and helping thousands of other people.

They break the post-Intro diet into five phases, when new things are systematically introduced, which is especially useful if your symptoms are severe. Their ebook, *SCD Lifestyle: From Surviving to Thriving*, is available at

http://scdlifestylebook.com

for $38. It's expensive for an ebook (they also include an audiobook version) but I found it worthwhile. I couldn't have figured out how to do SCD without it and their site. (*BTVC* helps you understand the science behind SCD, so both are valuable.) They have several other more expensive ebooks that I haven't purchased, including one very expensive course. I would prefer that all the material be available in one affordable book—they are frank about their intention to use internet marketing to become wealthy—but they also seem to have high integrity as well as good information. They are willing to answer emails, and if you have a tough problem, being pointed in the right direction can make all the difference.

Here's their page about celiac:

http://scdlifestyle.com/category/celiac-disease-series/

BREAKING THE VICIOUS CYCLE

http://www.breakingtheviciouscycle.info

is the official site for *BTVC*. The Legal/Illegal list and Knowledge Base are indispensable.

http://pecanbread.com

orients SCD toward children.

ALLISON SIEBECKER

http://www.siboinfo.com

focuses on SIBO. It's the site of Dr. Allison Siebecker, a naturopath who has made a specialty of it. She's working on a book about her SIBO Specific Diet, which combines SCD and low FODMAPS. Her podcasts are excellent.

http://tinyurl.com/SIBOFODMAP

is her chart that shows SCD legal foods from low to high FODMAPS.

An iOS app version is available:

http://tinyurl.com/qfbzczz

This is her summary of how to approach SIBO:

http://www.siboinfo.com/diet.html

There's some good big-picture material there.

JOHN BRISSON

Rather than our narrow focus on SIBO here, John has written a good comprehensive book covering all digestive disorders, including GERD, with many suggestions for supplement protocols and the pros and cons of various diets. His $7.99 Kindle book is here:

http://tinyurl.com/o3aqdnj

His site is here:

http://fixyourgut.com

GAPS

The GAPS diet is also based on SCD:

http://www.gapsdiet.com

The book about it is *Gut and Psychology Syndrome: Natural Treatment for Autism, Dyspraxia, A.D.D., Dyslexia, A.D.H.D., Depression, Schizophrenia*:

http://tinyurl.com/p2l45m7

OTHERS

These sites can lead you to a lot of other resources. Or do a web search for SCD. I'm not attempting here to tell you everything you need to know to successfully heal your gut. Health is complex. My aim is to present a framework so that you'll more quickly understand what you read elsewhere.

3 • WHAT DO YOU EAT?

Although SCD is restricted, there are plenty of delicious foods you can eat, and many great recipes, in *BTVC*, other books, and online, especially after you've been able to add back many of the gray-area foods. I'm not providing menu plans here because what each person can eat is so variable, but your meals can resemble a normal healthy diet minus the starches and sugars.

In later stages, you can have baked goods made with nut or coconut flours and honey to vary your diet or as a treat. Since working with unusual flours can be tricky, you might want to buy them already made.

http://www.scdbakery.com

… bakes fresh once a week and Priority mails out your order as soon as it's ready. It's expensive, but then, the ingredients are expensive and the recipes are labor-intensive. Every week, four products are available, and they change weekly. The recipes tend to use many of the same ingredients due to the restrictions of SCD, so the products tend to taste somewhat similar, but they are an enjoyable adjunct to the diet.

LEGAL/ILLEGAL

There are alphabetized lists online of what is legal and illegal on SCD. Here are two you can use to look up specific foods:

http://www.breakingtheviciouscycle.info/legal/listing/

http://www.pecanbread.com/p/legal_illegal_a-c.htm

But here are some generalizations:

Yes:

• Most non-starchy/ripe fresh fruits and vegetables, juices without sugar added and not from concentrate (sometimes sugar and chemicals are added to restore flavor; organic bottled concentrates are probably fine), some dried fruits in moderation
• Unprocessed meats, meat broths, unflavored gelatin
• Lactose-free milk products, such as hard cheese aged a month or more, homemade yogurt fermented twenty-four hours, and dry curd cottage cheese
• Eggs
• Plain nuts, coconut
• Some legumes, including lentils, peanuts, black beans, and navy beans
• Olives

No:

• Grains or grain-like seeds such as quinoa (you're eliminating all starches)
• Potatoes and yams
• Sweeteners except honey
• Processed foods, including most jarred and canned foods (Canned fish in only oil or water is okay. Tomato juice is fine. Elaine warns against other canned tomato products because sometimes illegal items are added but not disclosed; I've decided to trust organic products in moderation.)

• Mucilaginous foods such as okra, which are hard to digest

In More Detail

You might put this list in your phone, wallet, or purse. Here is an online version you can print:

https://shepherdhoodwin.com/scd/

SCD Legal:

<u>Meats</u>: eggs, chicken, turkey, beef, fish, pork, wild game, bacon, lamb

<u>Vegetables</u> (fresh or frozen): asparagus, beets, broccoli, Brussels sprouts, cabbage, cauliflower, carrots, celery, cucumbers, eggplant, garlic, kale, lettuce, mushrooms, onions, peas, peppers, pumpkin, spinach, squash, string beans, tomatoes, watercress

<u>Fruits</u> (fresh, frozen, or dried with nothing added): apples, avocados, bananas (ripe with black spots), berries, coconut, dates, grapefruit, grapes, kiwi, kumquats, lemons, limes, mangoes, melons, nectarines, oranges, papayas, peaches, pears, pineapples, prunes, raisins, rhubarb, tangerines

<u>Dairy</u>: SCD Yogurt, natural 30-day aged cheeses, butter, ghee, dry curd cottage cheese

<u>Nuts</u> (with no additives): almonds, pecans, Brazil, hazelnuts, walnuts, cashews, chestnuts

<u>Legumes</u>: peanuts, white/navy beans, lentils, split peas, lima beans, kidney beans, black beans

<u>Spices</u> (no anti-caking agents, all ingredients listed): most

<u>Drinks</u>: weak tea or coffee, water, mineral water, club soda, dry wine, gin, rye, scotch, bourbon, vodka
<u>Sweetener</u>: honey

SCD Illegal:

<u>Grains</u>: wheat, barley, corn, rye, oats, rice, buckwheat, millet, triticale, bulgur, spelt, quinoa
<u>Meats</u>: ham, processed sausages, lunch meats, bratwurst, turkey dogs, hot dogs
<u>Canned/Bottled Fruits, Vegetables, Juices</u> with added sugars, processing aids, preservatives
<u>Legumes</u>: soybeans, chickpeas, bean sprouts, mung beans, fava beans, garbanzo beans
<u>Dairy</u>: milk, commercial yogurts, unnatural/processed cheeses (Kraft, shredded, spreads, etc.), cottage, cream, feta, gjetost, mozzarella, Neufchatel, primost, ricotta
<u>Starches/tubers</u>: potatoes, yams, sweet potatoes, arrowroot, parsnip, cornstarch, tapioca starch
<u>Spices</u> with anti-caking agents: onion and garlic powders, blends such as curry (Simply Organic and Frontier are okay)
<u>Drinks</u>: instant coffee, most commercial juices, milk, soda pop, sweet wines, flavored liqueurs, brandy, sherry
<u>Sweeteners</u>: sugar of any kind (cane, coconut, table, etc.), agave, maple syrup, artificial sweeteners

FERMENTED FOODS

Fermented foods are great for healing the gut by implanting good bacteria to fight the bad, but their carriers may not be suitable for this diet. Kombucha, for example, is made with sugar, which is illegal.

Sauerkraut is made from cabbage (and other vegetables)—it's legal and perhaps the best probiotic food available, but cabbage is famously hard to digest, so caution is urged. I bought a container of raw sauerkraut, drained out the liquid to drink, and juiced the cabbage for the remaining good stuff. Raw sauerkraut is also easy to make if you add the liquid from a previous batch as a starter. Here are directions:

http://tinyurl.com/7mnx5vo

Bubbies is a company that makes some old-fashioned fermented foods with live cultures, including sauerkraut, dill pickles, and green tomatoes that have given superb results for some people with digestive issues. Read the labels, because some of their products have SCD-illegal sugar added. You want the products prepared without vinegar, indicating natural fermentation.

http://www.bubbies.com

For those who can handle dairy milk, SCD advocates a twenty-four-hour yogurt. Having a much longer fermentation time than normal yogurt, it uses up all the lactose, which is a disaccharide. The ingredients in commercial flavored yogurt are often appalling, and not all are disclosed on the labels. They also often include illegal ingredients such as pectin.

If you can't handle dairy milk, you can make it from nut or seed milks. Although whole nuts and especially seeds may be hard to handle at first, after blending them in fresh water for a long time, they are more broken down and should be okay in moderation. Soak and rinse whole nuts and seeds before making the milk in order to get rid of phytates, which are enzyme inhibitors that make them harder to digest. (Cashews are not technically nuts and don't need to be soaked, but a two-hour soak will make them blend more quickly.) An inexpensive nut milk bag or cheesecloth can be used to filter out sediment such as almond skins if you didn't blanch them first.

I got my non-dairy starter, GI ProStart, at

http://www.giprohealth.com

You can also use as a starter commercial plain yogurt as long as it doesn't have any illegal ingredients, but if you're going to be making a lot, you may as well invest in a real starter. In the long run, it will be cheaper than to keep buying commercial yogurt. It's not a good idea to use your old batch to start a new one more than once because bad bacteria can be introduced, unless you're using an heirloom starter, which can be found at

http://tinyurl.com/azsx3m2

Commercial starters have isolated bacterial strains, whereas heirloom starters have evolved structured communities that protect themselves against outside bacteria. They have been passed on for generations without degrading.

Bifidus is a probiotic often found in yogurt but it's illegal on SCD because it tends to take over.

Kefir is illegal because it is fermented with yeast as well as bacteria, and some lactose may remain.

Other normally healthy fermented foods such as miso and tamari are prohibited because soy is illegal, but again, I choose to use small amounts of organic, gluten-free varieties.

Kevita is a tasty sparkling probiotic drink that appears to be SCD legal and has some bacteria strains not found in other sources. If you like soda, this is a good substitute in small amounts, but carbonation in general is discouraged because it can cause bloating. Elaine allows one carbonated drink per week as long as it's free of illegal sweeteners.

Apple cider vinegar is allowed, but some vinegars aren't because they have sugar. I use organic brown rice vinegar; even though rice is illegal, by the time it's vinegar, no starch remains.

If you're not eating any probiotic foods, you'll want to take a good probiotic supplement. Even if you are, supplements may offer some strains of bacteria that you're not getting in your food. However, be sure to read the labels to check for SCD illegal additives such as inulin and maltodextrin. GI ProHealth offers an SCD legal probiotic with just acidophilus (also found in miso):

http://tinyurl.com/lpjddah

MAYONNAISE

Commercial mayonnaise has illegal ingredients. *BTVC* has a recipe for homemade mayonnaise in a food processor. I learned the hard way not to use olive oil, as it gets a metallic taste. Use a bland vegetable oil such as grape seed oil. Be sure to use only cold- or expeller-pressed oils; others use toxic chemicals to extract them.

4 • SHOPPING FOR THE DIET

ANTI-INFLAMMATORY TEA

It is helpful to drink a tea with turmeric, ginger, lemon, honey, coconut oil, and a dash of pepper two or three times a day. The usual way is to cut up fresh ginger and turmeric and boil it for several minutes, then strain and add honey and fresh-squeezed lemon juice.

To save time and money, I buy fresh ginger, turmeric, and lemons in bulk (about five pounds of each). I juice them and freeze the juice in one- or two-ounce squeeze bottles to use as needed. For best flavor, I use two squeezes each for the lemon and turmeric, and three for the ginger.

For the lemons, you'll need an inexpensive citrus juicer. I use a hand press. Some I've used have hurt my wrist after a while. This is by far the best one I've ever found:

https://tinyurl.com/uu2skbt

There are electric models as well, such as this one:

http://tinyurl.com/nq89rl4

For the ginger and turmeric, any vegetable juicer will work. This one is only $35:

http://tinyurl.com/l5muooo

A juicer that presses the pulp at a low temperature gives

you higher quality, longer-lasting juice. This is a well-reviewed single-gear model that is reasonably priced for its type:

https://tinyurl.com/t7oath2

The Green Star is a twin-gear model. It's sturdier and juicing is a little faster, but it's much more expensive:

http://tinyurl.com/klh5hsa

Both the gear juicers will juice wheatgrass.

You might find better prices on eBay.

After juicing the ginger and turmeric, I boil and strain the pulp three times, ending up with about a gallon of tea for each, which I use up before starting using the frozen juice.

I find raw unfiltered honey more delicious but *BTVC* says that clear pasteurized honey gives better results because the impurities in raw honey such as pollen might be irritating to the gut. It's a minor point but if your gut is in bad shape, every little bit helps. Costco has organic pasteurized honey in bears for a good price. Perhaps a better choice is their filtered raw wild honey, which shouldn't be irritating and has the health benefits and better flavor of being raw.

I found five pounds of organic fresh turmeric here for about $7/lb., about half the price local stores were selling it for:

http://tinyurl.com/mbq7f9s

I found commercial turmeric at a specialty supermarket

for about $4.50/lb.

Turmeric stains, so wear old clothes and keep everything in a small area for easier cleanup when juicing it. Add a dash of black pepper to your tea to make the curcumin (its active ingredient) in the turmeric far more bioavailable. Or drink it with food that contains pepper. Fat also makes the curcumin more bioavailable, so combine it with a tablespoon of coconut oil (whole turmeric also has some naturally occurring oil).

I got organic ginger for $3.50/lb. at a farmers market. I've found non-organic ginger for as little as $1/lb. at specialty supermarkets.

Commercial ginger generally shows low pesticide residues. I assume that that is also true of commercial turmeric. However, as with all commercial produce, I'd wash it with produce soap.

Costco sometimes has a five-pound bag of large organic lemons with twice as much juice as lemons I found elsewhere, and cheaper, too. Save some of the peels for lemon zest (the same with oranges and limes) for flavoring dishes, and add an eight of a peel to your smoothies—it has cancer-preventative properties. Trader Joe's usually has bags of smaller organic lemons for under $2/lb. Costco also carries an organic pasteurized lemon juice, "Italian Volcano," which is a big time- and money-saver, although it doesn't have the enzymes of raw lemons. Sometimes I substitute raw organic apple cider vinegar—it has great health benefits.

I bought the one-ounce flip-top plastic squeeze bottles here:

http://tinyurl.com/mcjoqmp

Two-ounce bottles are more convenient if you're drinking a lot of this tea, especially for ginger, since I use more of it, but I find the one-ounce size better for everyday use when not on SCD (I use raw ginger, lemon, and lime juices in smoothies, on salads, etc.) Find them here:

http://tinyurl.com/p5elhfl

Larger bottles are also available.

BONE BROTH

Bone broth is a welcome fad right now. Our ancestors routinely made rich bone broths to heal their guts. One source said that you will heal thirty percent faster if you include it abundantly in your diet (four to eight ounces, two or three times a day, is recommended). The reason is that simmering the bones for one to three days with a little apple cider vinegar in the water releases minerals and collagen that bathe your intestinal membranes in what they need. Bone broth is a staple of the GAPS diet, and is promoted by the Weston-Price Foundation and Sally Fallon in her excellent book *Nourishing Traditions*.

http://tinyurl.com/qfzd8pd

Unfortunately, its popularity means that bones (particularly beef) that you might have been able to get for next to nothing from a butcher in the past now are expensive. Organic, grass-fed beef marrow bones are

$6.50 a pound at my Whole Foods, and they're heavy! See if you can find a better deal at local butchers if you want to make it yourself. I'd go with at least grass-fed or organic if you can't get both. Beef bones should be simmered two or three days, poultry for one, and fish bones (which are tiny) for three hours.

http://www.wisechoicemarket.com

… has very high quality bone broth (both organic and grass-fed, in the case of beef), but it's pricey, about $17 for 24 ounces, shipped frozen on ice. They have both beef and chicken. The chicken is delicious, almost as good as homemade. Beef bone broth isn't as tasty, in my opinion, but it's okay, especially for cooking other foods. It's also good mixed with chicken broth.

Pacific Foods makes boxed organic chicken and turkey bone broths for about $5 a quart. Look for the word "bone" on the label; regular broth isn't mainly made from bones. It's more watery than the frozen broth from Wise Choice Market (the latter is thick enough to gel when it thaws) and isn't as tasty, but it's okay for the price, and sometimes goes on sale. If you want a stronger broth, you can simmer it without a lid to let some water evaporate. You can also flavor it with herbs and/or vegetables such as onions, celery, and carrots, and strain them out (onion and celery fiber can cause gas).

Golden Ladle brand is the best option for boxed chicken bone broth. It's organic, and thicker, tastier, and cheaper than Pacific Foods. Costco sometimes carries it for a very reasonable price. When they don't have it, their replacement isn't as good, but it is still probably the best price you'll find, and you can always add seasonings.

The cheapest option is to make fish broth from carcasses available free or cheap from a fish market (don't use oily fish). *Nourishing Traditions* advocates that. I did it once and will again. It's messy, smelly, and time consuming, but the meat I picked out of the head and fins was the richest, best fish I'd ever had. The broth is mild.

Beef, poultry, and fish broths each have different, equally beneficial healing properties, so it's good to do all three if you can, or at least poultry and beef.

A lot of SCD-legal foods can be simply prepared by boiling them in broth, making lovely simple soups. I like adding vegetable purees to bone broth to give rich, varied flavors, along with some meat and whole cooked vegetables such as squash.

Gelatin is also a good source of collagen and should be used liberally. In addition to gelled juices, I use it in my nut yogurt to make it firmer. You can also add it to smoothies. Sneak it in wherever you can. Here's a good one, kosher and made from grass-fed beef, at a good price:

http://tinyurl.com/jak4ve3

COSTCO

Costco is a godsend for this diet. In California, they have had, for example, ten-pound bags of excellent sweet organic carrots for under $5. You eat a lot of carrots on this diet in the beginning. SCD Lifestyle recommends boiling them for four hours but I've had good results just from steaming them for half an hour.

Sometimes I puree them (and other vegetables) in the steaming water.

Once, I found organic acorn squash at Costco for fifty cents a pound, also a great price. SCD Lifestyle suggests some elaborate, chef-level methods for preparing squash, but I just steam it and scoop it out (or peel the thin-skinned winter squashes with a carrot peeler). Rather than throwing away the seeds, I blend them for a long time in the steaming water and then strain it through a fine-mesh nut milk bag (you can use cheesecloth, too), making a savory seed milk that can be used as a soup base. Squash is a great food on this diet—it's filling and tasty, and has gentle fiber.

Cooked spinach is a pretty safe on SCD. Costco has a pound of fresh organic baby spinach for about $4. You can throw it into your soup at the end to wilt it. Cooking spinach lowers its oxalic acid, which inhibits absorption of nutrients. As mentioned, they also have other organic baby greens, including kale and a great salad mix.

Cooked, peeled apple and pear sauces are recommended early on by SCD. They're high FODMAP, so you might want to eat them alone. Costco is a good place for organic, high-quality fruit. (So is Sprouts Farmers Market.)

Bananas are allowed raw from the beginning—most people tolerate them well in moderation. Costco has three pounds of organic bananas for $2.

Their organic chicken is excellent and is $2.49/lb. It's free-range (I checked the brand's website). For my Intro diet, I boiled two whole ones in a stockpot for three hours along with carrots, onions, celery leaves, and parsley. Once it cooled, I took them out and strained the broth.

I removed the skin, fat, and bones from the meat, which I added back into the stock to simmer for another day along with some apple cider vinegar (which helps the bones leach healing minerals) to make bone broth. I stored a lot of the meat in four-ounce glass jelly jars (found in discount and hardware stores with canning jars) in the freezer for future use, keeping a large tub in the refrigerator to use during the Intro diet.

Onions are high FODMAP and can be hard to digest, and celery and parsley have tough fiber, so throw them away after straining the broth. (Save the carrots for pureeing.)

After straining the broth for the second time, let it cool overnight in the refrigerator, then skim off the fat. It's nutritious in moderation, but many people have trouble digesting fat and oil. You then assemble the soup, combining the broth with the chicken and pureed carrots.

You can cook down some of the broth to a delicious thick concentrate by letting it simmer with the lid off. A couple tablespoons added when heating up meats and vegetables adds flavor and moisture.

Jordan and Steve suggest using just breasts and thighs for the Intro Diet soup, which is more expensive than using the whole chicken. Adding chicken feet and backs (occasionally available at Whole Foods for about $3/lb.) gives you less usable meat but more bone broth. Costco and Trader Joe's have organic drumsticks, another alternative with a lot of bones, for $2/lb.

Costco also has organic ground beef at a great price (not grass-fed, though). However, I prefer their ground bison. It isn't labeled organic but it's better than non-organic beef because no growth hormones are used, and antibiotics aren't routinely used. Some comes from Australia, where it's likely one hundred percent grass-fed, but they have sources from three countries, so you have no way of knowing whether it's finished with grain. Since Costco sells things in large quantities (and I like saving time), I freeze it in four-ounce jars, taking out what I need to thaw a couple times a week.

Costco has two dozen organic eggs for slightly more than the price of one dozen organic eggs elsewhere. The label "free range" on eggs and chickens sold by chains simply means that the chickens have some, usually very limited, access to the outdoors and aren't kept in cages. For better-tasting eggs from chickens raised the old-fashioned way and from the heritage breeds, try farmers markets or someone with backyard chickens.

TRADER JOE'S

For the Intro diet, they recommend making gelatin with grape juice. TJ's has a quart of organic grape juice without sugar for $3.50 a bottle. I've made gelatin with other juices as well (diluted in half).

They also have organic Persian cucumbers, which are thin-skinned and seedless, and therefore easier to digest.

One of my staples is their frozen cod pieces, which is cheap, clean, sustainable, and from cold waters. It has a mild, neutral flavor.

CONDIMENTS

Most commercial condiments have illegal ingredients, but several products made for those on the Paleo diet are fine (if expensive)—read labels. For example, I'm a fan of barbecue sauce, and I found a Paleo version I like for about $6. I also improvised a quick substitute with a can of organic Costco tomato sauce, honey, apple cider vinegar, and a barbecue spice blend I bought in bulk from Sprouts.

Bubbies makes a relish with live probiotics.

5 • WAYS TO MAKE FOODS EASIER TO DIGEST

The thrust of this diet is to make digestion as easy as possible so that your small intestine can heal. Ways to make foods easier to digest include:

• Cook them well.

• Remove seeds, which are tough, for example, from zucchini and standard cucumbers.

• Use a blender, especially a high-speed blender such as a Vitamix, or a food processor S-blade to puree.

• Juice fruits and vegetables to remove the pulp.

• Only eat when you're peaceful. Stress is a known contributor to IBS (Irritable Bowel Syndrome).

• Chew everything well and eat slowly. Hold even juices in your mouth before swallowing them—don't gulp.

• Soak dried fruit to make them soft.

• Baby greens have less fiber (and more vitamins) than full-grown greens.

• Fermented foods are predigested.

• Take digestive enzymes and/or hydrochloric acid.

• Capsules are easier to digest than tablets. Large tablets sometimes gave me gut pain during my healing process. I tried soaking them in water, and some didn't break down even after long soaking—for higher potencies, sometimes manufacturers over-compress tablets—so I replaced them with capsules. It also might be better not to take too many supplements at once.

• Eat lightly at night. Especially for those with slow and compromised digestion, a heavy meal may not be fully digested by the time you go to bed, leading to gas and bloating. Furthermore, it is normal for digestion to be less vigorous later in the day. I find that I'm better off not eating meat after about 4 p.m.

• Soak raw whole nuts, seeds, beans, and grains (if/when you're eating them again later). Most are actually seeds, and their nature is to germinate. Soaking them in good water for a few hours to overnight (for beans) and then throwing away the water and rinsing them gets rid of phytates, nature's preservatives, and brings them to life. (Adding an acid such as lemon juice or vinegar, and a bit of salt, can help release them more effectively.) If you've soaked dry beans prior to cooking, you've seen how starchy the water is, and this diet eliminates starches. (Only some beans are SCD legal, and most of those are high FODMAP. Brown lentils are the best bet earlier on.)

Letting them go on to sprout (if they will) multiplies their nutrition and digestibility, although it changes their texture. I generally let beans (and grains, when not on SCD) sprout just slightly to minimize that, but a health blogger wrote that letting wheat sprout one-inch tails eliminated reactions in those with celiac (any longer than that, and bread made with ground up sprouts wouldn't hold together). *BTVC* says that those with celiac aren't actually reacting to the protein (gluten) but to the interaction of the protein with the carbohydrate. An experiment found that when the gluten was separated from the carbohydrate and then added back into bread, people didn't react to it. Apparently, that's what sprouting does.

• Observe good food combining principles. You're not eating any starch on SCD so you don't need to be concerned about combining it. The main thing is to eat fruit and honey alone, on an empty stomach, and wait until you've digested it (generally about thirty minutes) before a meal. If I have honey or a high-sugar fruit after a meal, my stomach instantly explodes from the fermentation.

I don't have a problem with combining greens with fruit in smoothies. The problem is combining sugar with heavier foods, especially animal products but also beans (nuts and seeds are okay). However, small amounts of papaya and pineapple, which have digestive enzymes, don't generally pose a problem. Neither do a few raisins or cranberries in a salad, or berries, which are low in sugar.

Although vegetables are considered to be a good combination with heavy foods, you might also want to eat high FODMAP vegetables such as asparagus, artichokes, cauliflower, and onions an hour before a heavier meal, since they, too, ferment quickly.

6 • SUPPLEMENTS

ANTIBIOTICS

Although diet alone can be successful in healing digestive disorders, you will probably need antibiotics (natural or pharmaceutical) to get rid of a bad case of SIBO, and they will speed up your healing in any case. To kill the bacteria overgrowth, try natural antibiotics first. If that doesn't work, you may need a pharmaceutical antibiotic such as Xifaxan (rifaximin is the generic name), which is stronger. As pharmaceutical antibiotics go, this one is relatively innocuous because it mostly targets the small intestine and doesn't do much damage to the flora in the colon.

The bacteria create a protective biofilm around themselves that also contains plastics, metals, and other toxins. Pharmaceutical antibiotics kill what's outside the film but not within, and then the bacteria can become more antibiotic resistant. After taking antibiotics, another hydrogen breath test might indicate that the bacteria is gone because what shows up is what's outside the biofilm, but the goal is to get through the biofilm so that the bacteria can truly and permanently die off.

Wade put me on antibiotic/antifungal supplements intended to penetrate increasingly deeper into the biofilm. The protocol is similar to this protocol for candida:

http://twjgifts.s3.amazonaws.com/Candida_Cleanse_Protocol.pdf

(Ignore the diet and skip to "Candida Cleanse

Supplements.")

It's best to be under the care of a holistic physician, naturopath, chiropractor, or nutritionist when attempting to solve a health problem as complex as SIBO. In addition, SIBO is often accompanied by other issues. If, for example, you also have an overgrowth of yeast such as candida, or parasites, you may need to get rid of it first before tackling the SIBO directly. Although there are similarities, the overall strategies for tackling candida and parasites are different than the one for SIBO. Also, if you're quite ill, you have to tread especially cautiously so as not to overwhelm your body; professional guidance can help you avoid costly mistakes.

In my protocol, I rotated five different supplements for four days at a time, completing a twenty-day cycle, two or three times total (forty or sixty days). They are: **pau d'arco** tea, **olive leaf** extract, **grapefruit seed** extract, **oregano** oil, and **Allicillin** (garlic, a trademarked form of allicin). The dose is three cups of pau d'arco a day, and four to eight capsules of the others. When using supplements that kill microbes, start with a lower dose and see how you're handling the die-off, which may have uncomfortable side effects. Gradually increase the dose to the maximum in order to overwhelm the microbes.

Instead of rotating every four days, Allison puts patients on four week courses of one to three of the following, at highest levels suggested on product label: allicin, oregano, neem, and cinnamon.

Practitioners more often recommend taking these with meals (like pharmaceutical antibiotics), but some recommend taking them between meals along with enzymes such as InterFase Plus that target the bacteria's biofilm (discussed below). There's no reason you couldn't do both—for example, four a day with meals in doses of two at a time, and four a day between meals with InterFase Plus, also in doses of two at a time.

Along with the rotating antibiotics, you can give the bacteria a one-two punch by taking **berberine**. In addition to being an excellent antibiotic for SIBO, it helps heal the mucous membrane of the small intestine. Wade likes Xymogen's Berbemycin:

http://tinyurl.com/lp4xven

Take three a day for twenty days with your rotating antibiotics.

A keystone of the protocol is **InterFase Plus** by Klaire Labs: "InterFase is a unique enzyme formulation especially designed to disrupt the biofilm matrix that embeds potential gastrointestinal pathogens." You start with two a day between meals and by the third week, increase it to eight, up to four at a time. In order to have it work on the bacteria and not act as a digestive aid, take it one to two hours before and after any food; first thing in the morning or even in the middle of the night is also fine. InterFase Plus is also a powerful healer for the small intestine and can be continued after completing the protocol above for a total of up to six months.

https://tinyurl.com/y83s65zj

There are other enzymes that help break down the

biofilm when taken between meals, such as carnivora (derived from venus flytrap) and bromelain (a common digestive enzyme when taken with food).

Another way to break down the biofilm is to drink a sludge first thing each morning containing a teaspoon of food-grade **diatomaceous earth** and a teaspoon of liquid **bentonite** clay (a half-teaspoon of each the first week). Wait half an hour before eating. In addition to bacteria, the silica in it is also metabolized by other microbes such as yeast, mold, fungi and parasites, killing them. Although my goal wasn't mainly to target yeast, this protocol is also used to combat candida and a good deal of yeast came out in my colonics. Diatomaceous earth also helps connect and build collagen as well as removing metals and microbial toxins. Since it can leach minerals, you can take a multi-mineral supplement.

The abrasive edges of the diatomaceous earth (silica is also what glass is made of) and the clay will leave your gut feeling less settled. You need to learn to differentiate between the unsettling from it and a food reaction. Although the point of SCD is to calm the intestines, the collateral damage of this protocol is worth it because you can't heal your small intestine until you get rid of the bacteria overgrowth. No matter how you do it, there will be irritation—there's no way around that. Once the bacteria is under control, you can focus on healing the intestinal membrane through SCD, bone broth, probiotics, and other supplements.

Take the diatomaceous earth for four weeks, and wait a year before doing another round. You can continue with the bentonite, since it absorbs toxins and can also help clean the large intestine.

Diatomaceous earth:

http://tinyurl.com/kkthvt4

Bentonite:

http://tinyurl.com/mpdgkz4

Before bed, I take four **saccharomyces boulardii**, a yeast-eating strain of probiotic. I got a cheap, well-reviewed one at Swanson:

http://tinyurl.com/puvkkzm

It may seem counterintuitive to take probiotics while trying to get rid of bacterial overgrowth, and it's true that efforts to repopulate your gut with good bacteria will be more successful once you're done eliminating the overgrowth. However, it is useful to take probiotics and/or eat fermented probiotic foods even while working to kill the bacteria overgrowth because they increase the proportion of good to bad bacteria—the good bacteria keep the bad in check. Wait an hour after taking an antibiotic before taking probiotics.

A quick web search shows a number of other natural remedies for SIBO, including food grade peppermint oil, raw garlic, neem, coconut oil, golden seal, cat's claw, and cinnamon. Primal Defense Ultra by Garden of Life contains bacillus subtilis, which one poster said, "annihilates bacteria. It is really quite amazing." Aloe vera is illegal on SCD—it's mucilaginous and an immune booster—but one commenter found a brand, Ultimate Aloe Vera, to be helpful; it's processed in such a way that it doesn't have a laxative effect. (It's quite expensive.)

REBUILDING THE GUT

After knocking out the SIBO, your focus shifts to rebuilding the small intestinal membrane. Diet and bone broth are your main approaches, but some supplements can help. John Brisson (https://www.fixyourgut.com) recommends L-glutamine, N-acetyl glucosamine (NAG), and curcumin (from turmeric), although if you're drinking the tea with fresh turmeric, you're probably covered on that. He also recommends strong probiotics, which might be covered if you're making yogurt and raw sauerkraut, but couldn't hurt. B vitamins are important throughout your healing process, especially B-12.

HCL and DIGESTIVE ENZYMES

As we age, we produce less hydrochloric acid and fewer digestive enzymes.

Low stomach acid (including from the use of antacids) is one cause of SIBO, because hydrochloric acid kills excess bacteria. Wade recommended HCL Activator:

http://tinyurl.com/l33squ7

It works well with Premier HCL:

http://tinyurl.com/onl7l9d

You take both after meals.

Raw foods contain enzymes that are destroyed with cooking. Especially since you don't eat much raw food when you first start SCD, digestive enzymes help you digest your food more efficiently, allowing your small intestine to better rest and heal. It's a good idea to take them with all cooked food. Some enzymes target fats, others proteins, and others carbs. If you know you have trouble with digesting, say, protein, you can load up on the relevant enzymes. There are many good formulas that combine all three. This is what I take with meals:

http://tinyurl.com/p4f85o5

SOLE

A good, inexpensive source of minerals is Himalayan sea salt. You can make "sole" by soaking a salt chunk in distilled water until it is saturated, about twenty-four hours, and take one teaspoon a day. This is said to be more potent than simply using the salt on food. Here is a good source:

http://tinyurl.com/lcjhv8a

OTHER SUPPLEMENTS

SCD recommends various supplements that may be important to its success, such as Vitamins C and D, and a B complex.

http://www.giprohealth.com

… has some supplements specifically for people doing SCD.

In general, I find the best prices and selection on supplements (and some foods, too) at

http://www.vitacost.com

In second place is

http://www.swansonvitamins.com

Both have great sales and coupons (get on their email lists).

I also find some things at Amazon.

KEEPING TRACK OF SUPPLEMENTS, ETC.

It is complicated to keep track of what to take and when. I created a simple table in Microsoft Word that lists all the things I'm taking so that I don't forget. I write down the times in the boxes. On the left is the day/date. Since I'm rotating the antifungals/ antibiotics, I entered their names to remind myself of which one I'm supposed to take each day.

Here is a PDF online you can print:

https://tinyurl.com/yblh52bt

SIBO

Day/Date	Diatomaceous Bentonite	Oil Pulling	B12	Salt Gargle	Tea: Turmeric Ginger, etc.	Broth	InterFase	Antifungals	Supplements
W19								PAU	
H20									
F21									
S22									
Su23								OLV	
M24									
U25									
W25									
H27								GRPFRT	
F28									
S29									
Su3/1									
M2								ORGNO	
U3									
W4									
H5									
F6								ALLCN	

7 • REDUCING TOXINS

WATER FILTERING

Since reducing toxins in your body (and your immune response to them) is a goal of this protocol, consider filtering your water or installing a reverse osmosis system under your kitchen sink (relatively inexpensive systems are available at Amazon and Costco). Reverse osmosis is the most effective way to remove toxins from tap water, but it also removes beneficial minerals along with heavy metals, so be sure to add minerals back in. This is a good product for that:

http://tinyurl.com/ncjnwva

You can also use sole, mentioned above.

Just as important is having a shower filter to eliminate chlorine. This is a good one because it gets out more than just chlorine:

http://tinyurl.com/kc2eyod

Elaine also recommends avoiding chlorinated pools and spas.

BUY ORGANIC

Buying organic whenever you can is a good idea. If not, there are natural unscented soaps that can wash insecticides off produce. You don't need to buy a dedicated produce wash, since they're much more expensive. Shaklee's Basic H is a good product for this purpose:

http://www.shaklee.com

At local farmers markets in Southern California, most vendors say that their produce is free of pesticides and chemical fertilizers but aren't certified organic because it's too expensive for them to get certified. That's good enough for me. Even chemical fertilizers don't bother me much—it's the sprays that are most dangerous. Fortunately, in dry climates like California, insects aren't a big problem and sprays are often unnecessary. If you must buy non-organic, look for California-grown vs. Florida-grown, since far more pesticides need to be used in that humid climate.

Here are the "CLEAN 15" fruits and vegetables that are generally low in insecticides and therefore safe to buy non-organic (often due to having a thick skin that you're not going to eat). I edited out those that are not SCD legal:

Avocados, pineapples, cabbage, sweet peas (frozen), onions, asparagus, mangoes, papayas, kiwi, eggplant, grapefruit, cantaloupe (domestic), cauliflower.

These are the "DIRTY DOZEN," which should be bought organic (again edited):

Apples, strawberries, grapes, celery, peaches, spinach, peppers, nectarines (imported), cucumbers, cherry tomatoes, snap peas (imported), blueberries (domestic).

I also included these lists here:

https://shepherdhoodwin.com/scd/

Consumer Reports breaks it down by country. For example, commercial winter squash from Guatemala has a very low pesticide risk whereas U.S. grown has a high risk.

FRUITS: https://tinyurl.com/ydfucov3
VEGETABLES: https://tinyurl.com/ydyray75

The most vital foods to be organic are animal products, since they are higher on the food chain and their toxins are in greater concentration. In addition, organic eggs have a healthy ratio of omega-6 to omega-3 essential fatty acids whereas commercial eggs do not. If you tolerate milk, raw products are healthier.

Although fish is highly nutritious, our overfished, polluted waters make it problematic. SUSTAINABLE fish (not in danger of being overfished) include salmon, snapper, mahi, cod, and chard. LOW MERCURY seafood includes shrimp, sardines, scallops, and oysters. Smaller fish like sardines and anchovies are less contaminated in general because they are lower on the food chain. Wild fish (versus farmed) is also generally cleaner, although farmed shellfish such as scallops are okay. Cold water fish such as cod and salmon are high in omega-3 fatty acids. You can find longer lists online. These are also here:

https://shepherdhoodwin.com/scd/

BATHS

Soaking in a tub with various substances added can help you detoxify. The skin is our largest elimination organ. You can add any combination of sea salt, mineral salts, Epsom salt, hydrogen peroxide, various healing essential oils, ginger, baking soda, bentonite clay, seaweed, apple cider vinegar, and more. A web search will give you more information.

Good essential oils for detoxification include peppermint, juniper, grapefruit, rosemary, laurel, mandarin, lemon oil, patchouli, hyssop, and helichrysum.

For relaxation and other benefits, try rose, cedarwood, sandalwood, rosewood, neroli, vetiver, lavender, chamomile, ylang ylang, or jasmine.

If you mix essential oils in a carrier oil such as olive, jojoba, or almond oil before adding them to your bath water, they are less likely to evaporate or burn your skin.

OIL PULLING

Oil pulling is a folk remedy for detoxing. It's beneficial for both your dental health and your whole body. It's covered here:

http://en.wikipedia.org/wiki/Oil_pulling

Best results are from raw, organic coconut oil, which also kills many microbes. (You can brush your teeth with it, too, combined with baking soda.) High quality olive or sesame oil can also be used. Cheap processed oils aren't recommended, since you'll absorb some.

Adding healing essential oils can increase its benefits; rotating a variety of them is best. Some good choices are birch (great for treating tooth decay), rosemary, peppermint, oregano, tea tree, myrrh, frankincense, geranium, grapefruit, lemon, lemongrass, and orange. Clove and cinnamon are good for tooth pain.

Here is a good source for one hundred percent pure essential oils (some brands are not meant for internal use and are adulterated):

http://www.edensgarden.com

TOILET STOOL

If you sit on the toilet using a stool with your legs bent, approximating the natural squatting position, you'll have easier and more thorough eliminations. Here's a good toilet stool:

http://tinyurl.com/qaf5dkt

ENEMAS AND COLONICS

Many people have layers of mucoid plaque lining their colon wall, built up from years of eating SAD—the Standard American Diet filled with overly refined and junk foods. Cleansing the colon can contribute greatly to health. The products by Arise & Shine are the gold standard:

http://ariseandshine.com

The basic approach is to use herbs to loosen the plaque, and psyllium seed husks and bentonite clay to sweep it out. Psyllium is illegal on SCD (it's too rough, for one thing), but it might be a good idea to do a full colon cleanse including colonic hydrotherapy once you've tamed your SIBO and healed your small intestine.

In the meantime, however, when you're detoxing, a lot of the poisons end up in your large intestine and need to be carried out of your body so that you don't reabsorb some of them. For most of us, our elimination isn't as effective as it might be. Colonics can help get rid of what you're not otherwise eliminating.

There are two kinds of colonics: the older closed system, which is administered by the therapist, letting in water, and then letting it out with the waste. Five to ten gallons of water are typically used. I prefer the open system, in which you're basically perched over a horizontal toilet and water comes in and out continuously, up to twenty-five gallons. It's more do-it-yourself, and I find that it can be a deeper cleanse—more comes out. However, I've also had good success with closed-system colonics—it depends on the specific equipment and practitioner.

For a couple days prior to your colonic, avoid gas-producing foods such as beans, broccoli, cauliflower, cabbage, onions, cucumbers, carrots, raw apples, and bananas. Otherwise, your colonic will be devoted largely to getting rid of the gas. Afterward for a day or more, avoid raw vegetables and have soft, warm foods such as soups and pureed cooked vegetables so that your colon can recover and rebalance. Take probiotics to add back what you eliminated.

In my area (Orange County, California), colonics cost $75-90, which is pricey, especially since you'll probably want to have more than one, particularly when you're not having good eliminations on your own. Some places offer a deal for new clients, such as half price for the first three, or a discounted package. You might also find a coupon online; I found a Groupon for three colonics for $90 with an open system.

A friend who had already been living a healthy lifestyle went to a holistic clinic to have a ten-day water fast (eating no food, and drinking only water). Part of the package was a daily colonic. On the ninth day, nothing had come out. On the tenth, he considered skipping it, but since he'd already paid for it and having nothing to lose, he was persuaded to do it. Suddenly, a torrent of pitch-black crud came pouring out of him. He almost floated out of his body in kundalini ecstasy, which lasted three days. The colonic had probably finally reached the final third of the large intestine, the ascending colon, which is hardest to reach with colonics. Who knows what we're carrying around in us that could show up later in life as a disease? It's best to stay as clean internally as possible.

If you can't do colonics, home enemas can be helpful, although they aren't nearly as thorough. There are various kinds besides using plain water. Coffee enemas aren't about cleansing the colon, but of detoxifying the liver. They are very useful for a variety of conditions, and are safe if you use common sense. I have a friend who gets high from them. I haven't had that experience, but whenever you release something that's been holding you down, it's going to feel great. We joked that we should start a chain of coffee shops called Starf*cks, with hoses of gourmet coffee you can plug into your butt. My friend recommends using whole green coffee beans boiled in water for an hour (always use organic), although traditionally, standard ground coffee is used. Do them early in the day in case the caffeine affects you, but after a good bowel movement so you can hold in the coffee water for fifteen minutes without discomfort. You can find full instructions online.

ABOUT THE AUTHOR

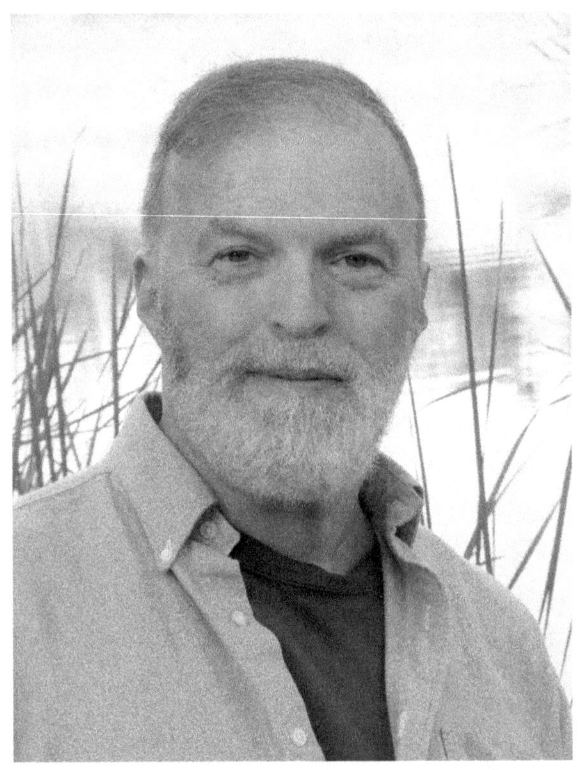

SHEPHERD HOODWIN has been channeling since 1986. He also does intuitive readings, mediumship, past-life regression, healing, counseling, and channeling coaching (teaching others to channel). He has conducted workshops on the Michael teachings throughout the United States and Europe.

Shepherd is a graduate of the University of Oregon. He lives in Laguna Niguel, California.

ABOUT THE AUTHOR

https://shepherdhoodwin.com

TWITTER:
@shepherdh
@EnlightenNitwit

FACEBOOK:
https://www.facebook.com/shepherd.hoodwin
https://www.facebook.com/shepherd.hoodwin.author/
https://www.facebook.com/JourneyOfYourSoul/
https://www.facebook.com/EnlightenmentforNitwits/

shepherdhoodwin@gmail.com

Summerjoy Press
99 Pearl
Laguna Niguel CA 92677-4818

OTHER BOOKS BY SHEPHERD HOODWIN

Available at https://shepherdhoodwin.com/book/

All Is Choice

Few realize how profound, multi-faceted, and far-reaching the concept of choice is in our spiritual growth. This short book explores topics such as what is and is not our right to choose, our power as creators and the limits of our reality creation, how consciousness expands, and much more. Being in the World

This insightful book explores practical spirituality. Topics include aging, karma, time, and religion.

Being in the World

This insightful book explores practical spirituality. Topics include aging, karma, time, and religion.

Compassion for Evil
A Metaphysical View

Compassion for Evil explores the nature of evil from the soul's point of view, and how we can skillfully deal with it as lightworkers.

Embracing What Is
Spiritual Keys to Happiness

This book is an abridged version of *Happiness and the Michael Teachings*, without technical Michael teachings terminology. A free version is available at Smashwords.com.

Energy Literacy
How to Perceive and Take Charge of Your Spiritual Well-Being

Energy Literacy is an introduction to how to perceive our energy field and release negativity. Topics include chakras, contracts, vows, cording, entities, implants, psychic attack, earthbound souls, soul retrieval, and more.

Enlightenment for Nitwits
The Complete Guide

This hilarious metaphysical/self-help humor collection will appeal to Oprah and Dave Barry fans as well as those with more esoteric interests. In a style reminiscent of comedian Steven Wright, it's full of wry one-liners along with longer, hilariously mind-bending pieces on a wide range of subjects, tied together by the idea of clueless humans trying to find enlightenment.

"I love _Enlightenment for Nitwits_! It is the funniest book I have read in several decades. If laughter leads to enlightenment, it will certainly do it. Nothing—thank God—is sacred in this delightful spoof on life in general."
—C. Norman Shealy, M.D., author of _Life Beyond 100_

Growing Through Joy
This thought-provoking book explores the nature of

personal growth.

Happiness and the Michael Teachings
Learning to Embrace What Is
Happiness is the ultimate goal of every spiritual teaching. Here we explore several principles of what the Michael teachings refer to as growing through joy.

Journey of Your Soul
A Channel Explores the Michael Teachings
This is the most in-depth discussion of the Michael teachings to date. It may also be the first analytical study of channeling written by a channel. It has forewords by John Friedlander, author of *Psychic Psychology*, and Jon Klimo, author of *Channeling: Investigations on Receiving Information from Paranormal Sources*. Klimo writes, "*Journey of Your Soul* may well be the best (Michael) book of them all due to its clarity, thoroughness, and detail, and thanks to the fact that the author, an exceptionally clear-headed Michael channel himself, brings real integrity and authenticity to our understanding of Michael in particular and to the channeling process in general."

Loving from Your Soul
Creating Powerful Relationships

This inspiring, transformative book explores the nature of love itself as well as practical matters of relationships. One reader wrote, "There are phrases that are so inspiring that I wrote them down to refer to when I need them. I am looking forward to reading this book again and again."

Meditations for Self-Discovery
Guided Journeys for Communicating with Your Inner Self

This is a beautiful collection of forty-five vivid, often pastoral, guided imagery meditations channeled from Shepherd's essence. There are many meditation recordings available, but this is one of the first collections of meditations in book form that can be read to oneself or others. Teachers and group leaders would find it particularly useful.

Opening to Healing

This uplifting book explores the spiritual aspect of healing.

Unconditional Love in Politics
Or Have You Hugged a Republican/Democrat Today?

Is unconditional love in politics an oxymoron? Thus far, it's been a rare commodity if it's ever been there. This book explores what you can do about it, as well as why both right and left have useful parts to play in our evolution, the factors that influence a person's tilt to the right or left, and what unconditional love might look like in this sphere.

Why We're Attracted
Spiritual, Psychological and Physical Elements That Draw Us to Others

Just why are we attracted to some people and not to others? This book explores a multitude of factors on three levels: spiritual, psychological, and physical. Topics include agreements, life path, soul chemistry, male/female energy ratio, celibacy, body-type attraction, sexual orientation, monogamy, and polyfidelity.

At last, a practical, useful guide. I like that the author shares his experiences as well as solutions and helpful buying resources. Thank you!

Well written, great information.

Very great reference! This book is so helpful and loaded with information. I am also pleased to see all the links available.

Last week I was on a beach holiday and dealing with the extreme bloating that is so common for me even after eating just small amounts.

I added this to my Kindle a few months ago and finally was ready to read it all. I'm so grateful for this information!

I've had stomach problems and general poor gut issues since I was six. Now I'm nearly forty and want to finally get well! The information in this book is really helpful. It's written well and the tone is like having an in-depth conversation with a very knowledgeable friend who gets it and sincerely wants me to experience wellness. He shares lots of good links to learn more about the Specific Carbohydrate Diet (SCD) and has inspired me to finally heal my gut for good.

Reading this is time well spent.